AUTOIMMUNE PROTOCOL JUICING COOKBOOK

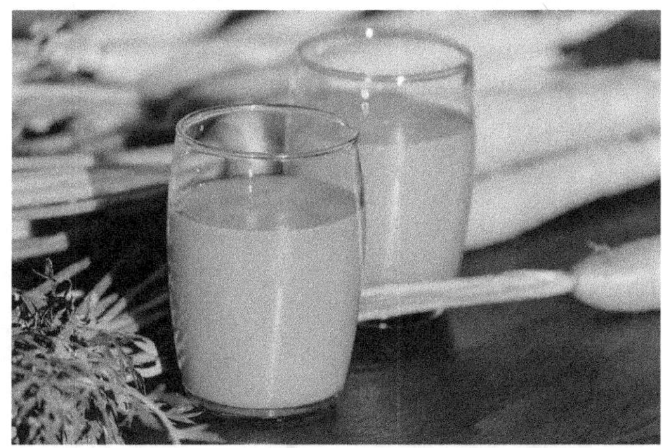

DR. MAUREEN MOORE

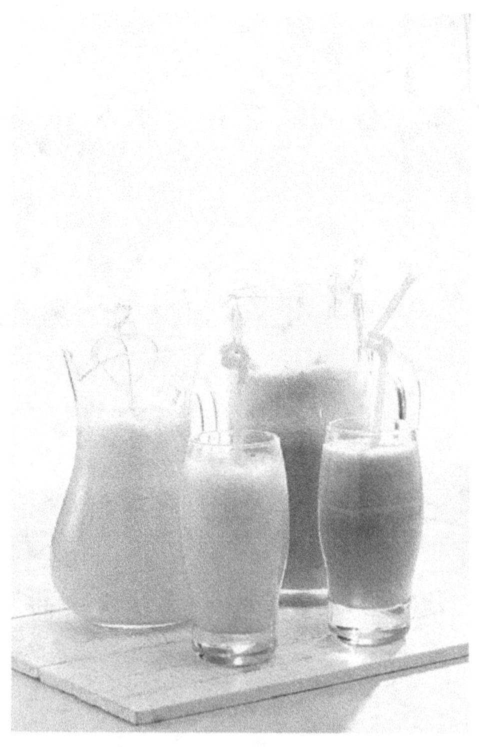

TABLE OF CONTENT

CHAPTER ONE 7

How to use autoimmune protocol....................7

Juicing cookbook 7

Understanding Autoimmune Protocol Juicing..10

Principles of Autoimmune Protocol Juicing.....11

Benefits of Autoimmune Protocol Juicing........13

Tips on Autoimmune Protocol Juicing 16

Guidelines of Autoimmune Protocol Juicing ...18

CHAPTER TWO...22

Autoimmune Protocol Juicing Recipes 22

1. Berry Citrus Blast 22

2. Green Apple Ginger Zinger 23

3. Pineapple Turmeric Sunrise.....................24

4. Mango Mint Cooler 25

5. Carrot Apple Cinnamon Elixir..................25

6. Beet Berry Bliss 26

7. Papaya Lime Refresher 27

8. Blueberry Kale Kickstart 28

9. Orange Carrot Ginger Energizer 29

10. Melon Mint Hydration Splash 30

11. Cucumber Avocado Green Goddess 31

12. Tomato Basil Bliss...................................32

13. Sweet Potato Coconut Elixir 33

14. Broccoli Lemon Zest Delight 34

15. Butternut Squash Sage Elixir....................35

16. Asparagus Cilantro Citrus Blend 35

17. Spinach Pineapple Mint Fusion.................36

18. Cauliflower Rosemary Elixir.....................37

19. Zucchini Basil Green Refresher 38

20. Bell Pepper Carrot Turmeric Elixir 39

21. Turmeric Cauliflower Delight 40

22. Spinach Avocado Green Elixir 41

23. Carrot Ginger Butternut Soup...................42

24. Zucchini Broccoli Basil Elixir...................43

25. Tomato Bell Pepper Herb Elixir.................44

26. Cabbage Carrot Apple Fusion....................44

27. Beet Berry Basil Elixir............................45

28. Spinach Cucumber Mint Cooler.................46

29. Bell Pepper Carrot Ginger Elixir...............47

30. Broccoli Kale Lemon Zest Elixir 48

31. Berry Coconut Chia Pudding.....................49

32. Cucumber Guacamole Cups 50

33. Sweet Potato Kale Chips 51

34. Apple Cinnamon Collagen Bites 52

35. Beet Hummus with Veggie Sticks 53

36. Turmeric Almond Energy Bites.................54

37. Avocado Basil Zoodles 55

8. Pineapple Mint Popsicles.................................56

9. Cabbage Wrap with Turkey and Avocado 56

10. Mango Tango Salsa with Jicama 57

CONCLUSION 59

CHAPTER ONE

Understand the Basics:

Begin by familiarizing yourself with the autoimmune protocol (AIP) and its principles. The AIP diet is designed to reduce inflammation and support those with autoimmune conditions. Gain insights into the foods to include and avoid in your diet.

Get the Right Ingredients:

Stock your kitchen with AIP-friendly ingredients. This may include fresh vegetables, fruits, lean proteins, healthy fats, and herbs. Ensure you have a variety of colorful and nutrient-dense options that align with the AIP guidelines.

Explore the Cookbook:

Take a thorough look at your Autoimmune Protocol Juicing Cookbook. Pay attention to the introduction, which often provides insights into the AIP, juicing benefits, and tips on how to maximize the recipes for your health goals.

Meal Planning: Plan your meals in advance. Consider incorporating the juicing recipes into your weekly meal plan. This will help you stay organized, ensure a diverse range of nutrients, and make your AIP journey more sustainable.

Start with Simple Recipes:

Begin your juicing journey with simple recipes. Look for basic combinations that align with your taste preferences and gradually experiment with more complex blends as you become accustomed to the flavors.

Follow Serving Sizes:

Pay attention to serving sizes in the cookbook. While the ingredients are nutritious, moderation is key. Following the recommended portion sizes ensures a balanced intake of nutrients without overdoing it.

Listen to Your Body:

Everyone's body responds differently, so pay attention to how your body reacts to specific ingredients. If you notice any adverse reactions or sensitivities, adjust your recipes accordingly.

Experiment with Flavors:

Don't be afraid to experiment with flavors. Mix and match ingredients to find combinations that appeal to your taste buds. This not only keeps your meals exciting but also encourages adherence to the AIP lifestyle.

Stay Hydrated:

Hydration is crucial in any health-focused journey. Incorporate hydrating elements into your juices, such as cucumber or coconut water. Adequate hydration supports overall well-being and helps flush out toxins.

Seek Professional Guidance:

If you have specific health concerns or dietary restrictions, consider consulting with a healthcare professional or a nutritionist. They can provide personalized advice and ensure that the AIP juicing recipes align with your individual health needs.

Remember, the Autoimmune Protocol Juicing Cookbook is a tool to support your well-being. Enjoy the process of discovering new flavors, nourishing your body, and embracing a lifestyle that contributes to your overall health and vitality.

Understanding Autoimmune Protocol Juicing

Understanding the Autoimmune Protocol (AIP) Juicing involves delving into a dietary approach designed to manage autoimmune conditions by mitigating inflammation and promoting overall well-being.

The AIP emphasizes the elimination of potential trigger foods, focusing on nutrient-dense options that support immune function and gut health.

In the context of juicing, this protocol translates into creating beverages that harness the healing power of fruits, vegetables, and herbs while avoiding ingredients that could exacerbate autoimmune responses.

The cornerstone of AIP juicing is the incorporation of anti-inflammatory and nutrient-rich ingredients. This may include leafy greens, berries, turmeric, ginger, and other foods renowned for their healing properties.

By emphasizing a diverse array of fruits and vegetables, AIP juicing aims to provide essential vitamins, minerals, and antioxidants crucial for immune modulation.

Moreover, the AIP Juicing approach recognizes the importance of eliminating potential allergens or irritants, such as nightshades and certain spices, which could trigger autoimmune reactions.

It encourages a mindful exploration of ingredients, promoting a personalized approach based on individual sensitivities and health goals.

In essence, AIP Juicing is a holistic strategy that combines the principles of the Autoimmune Protocol with the therapeutic potential of freshly pressed juices, creating a flavorful and health-supportive union tailored to those navigating autoimmune challenges.

Principles of Autoimmune Protocol Juicing

The principles of Autoimmune Protocol (AIP) Juicing are rooted in the belief that dietary choices play a pivotal role in managing autoimmune conditions by addressing inflammation and supporting overall health.

The following key principles guide the AIP Juicing approach:

Anti-Inflammatory Focus: AIP Juicing centers around ingredients known for their anti-inflammatory properties. Leafy greens, cruciferous vegetables, and berries are often staples, as they contain compounds that may help mitigate inflammation, a common feature in autoimmune disorders.

Nutrient Density: The emphasis is on nutrient-dense foods to provide a broad spectrum of essential vitamins, minerals, and antioxidants. AIP Juicing seeks to optimize nutritional intake to support immune function and overall well-being.

Elimination of Potential Triggers: The AIP diet identifies and eliminates potential trigger foods that might exacerbate autoimmune responses. This includes commonly inflammatory foods such as nightshades, grains, and certain spices, promoting a cautious and personalized approach to ingredient selection.

Gut Health Support: AIP Juicing recognizes the crucial role of gut health in autoimmune conditions. Ingredients like bone broth and probiotic-rich foods may be incorporated to nurture a healthy gut microbiome, fostering immune balance.

Mindful Ingredient Selection: Individuals are encouraged to be mindful of their body's responses to different ingredients. AIP Juicing promotes self-awareness and customization, acknowledging that each person's tolerance and sensitivities may vary.

Holistic Wellness: Beyond managing autoimmune conditions, AIP Juicing aligns with the broader principles of holistic wellness. It encourages a lifestyle that encompasses stress management, adequate sleep, and regular physical activity to support overall health.

By adhering to these principles, AIP Juicing seeks to empower individuals to make informed dietary choices that align with their health goals and contribute to a balanced and nourishing lifestyle.

Benefits of Autoimmune Protocol Juicing

The benefits of Autoimmune Protocol (AIP) Juicing extend beyond the refreshing taste of vibrant concoctions to encompass a spectrum of health advantages tailored for individuals navigating autoimmune challenges.

Reduced Inflammation: AIP Juicing prioritizes anti-inflammatory ingredients such as turmeric, ginger, and leafy greens. These components may assist in reducing inflammation, a key factor in many autoimmune conditions.

Nutrient Optimization: By focusing on nutrient-dense fruits and vegetables, AIP Juicing provides a concentrated source of vitamins, minerals, and antioxidants. This nutrient optimization supports overall health and aids the body's natural healing processes.

Gut Health Enhancement: AIP Juicing incorporates ingredients like bone broth and probiotic-rich foods, promoting a healthy gut microbiome.

Improved Digestive Function: Juicing facilitates the pre-digestion of nutrients, easing the burden on the digestive system. For individuals with autoimmune conditions affecting the gastrointestinal tract, this can provide relief and support improved nutrient absorption.

Energy Boost: The influx of essential nutrients and hydration from AIP Juicing may contribute to increased energy levels.

This is particularly beneficial for individuals with autoimmune disorders who often experience fatigue as a common symptom.

Hydration Support: Many AIP Juicing recipes incorporate hydrating ingredients like cucumber and coconut water, supporting optimal hydration. Proper hydration is crucial for overall health and can positively impact various bodily functions.

Weight Management: AIP Juicing can be a valuable component of a holistic approach to weight management. By focusing on nutrient-dense, whole foods, individuals may experience better control over their weight, a factor relevant to autoimmune conditions.

Antioxidant Defense: AIP Juicing harnesses the power of antioxidants found in fruits and vegetables, helping to neutralize free radicals and protect cells from oxidative stress. This antioxidant defense is particularly important in managing autoimmune conditions.

Incorporating AIP Juicing into a wellness routine offers a multifaceted approach to support individuals dealing with autoimmune challenges.

From reducing inflammation to enhancing gut health and providing a nutrient-rich boost, the benefits extend beyond the glass, fostering a holistic sense of well-being.

Tips on Autoimmune Protocol Juicing

Embarking on the Autoimmune Protocol (AIP) Juicing journey requires a thoughtful approach to maximize its benefits while accommodating individual needs and sensitivities. Here are essential tips to enhance your AIP Juicing experience:

Consult with a Healthcare Professional: Before adopting AIP Juicing, especially if managing autoimmune conditions, consult with a healthcare professional or a registered dietitian. They can provide personalized guidance based on your specific health status.

Gradual Introduction: Introduce AIP Juicing gradually to allow your body to adapt. Sudden dietary changes may impact some individuals differently, so observe how your body responds to each new ingredient.

Diversify Ingredients: Aim for diversity in your juices by incorporating a wide range of fruits, vegetables, and herbs.

This not only provides a spectrum of nutrients but also prevents monotony in taste.

Mindful Ingredient Selection: Be mindful of the AIP principles by excluding potential trigger foods. Avoid nightshades, grains, dairy, and other ingredients that might elicit autoimmune responses.

Monitor Sugar Content: While fruits contribute natural sweetness, be cautious with high-sugar fruits to manage sugar intake. Opt for lower-sugar options and balance sweetness with savory elements.

Include Healing Herbs: Incorporate herbs like turmeric and ginger, known for their anti-inflammatory properties. These additions not only enhance flavor but also contribute to the therapeutic benefits of AIP Juicing.

Hydrate Adequately: Complement AIP Juicing with sufficient water intake. Hydration is essential for overall health and helps flush out toxins.

Experiment with Texture: Explore different textures by blending or juicing to find what suits your preferences. Smoothies with added fiber can provide a more satiating experience.

Listen to Your Body: Pay attention to how your body reacts to specific ingredients. If you notice any adverse effects, adjust your recipes accordingly. Your body's responses can guide you in tailoring AIP Juicing to your individual needs.

Combine with Balanced Meals: AIP Juicing is most effective when integrated into a balanced and varied diet.

By approaching AIP Juicing with these tips in mind, you can create a customized and enjoyable experience that aligns with the principles of autoimmune health, fostering wellness from within.

Guidelines of Autoimmune Protocol Juicing

Following guidelines for Autoimmune Protocol (AIP) Juicing ensures a structured and health-supportive approach to managing autoimmune conditions. Here are essential guidelines to consider:

Understand AIP Principles: Familiarize yourself with the core principles of the Autoimmune Protocol. This includes eliminating potential trigger foods like nightshades, grains, and dairy.

Consult with a Professional: Seek guidance from a healthcare professional or a registered dietitian familiar with autoimmune conditions. They can provide personalized advice based on your health status.

Prioritize Nutrient-Dense Ingredients: Emphasize nutrient-dense fruits and vegetables to maximize the therapeutic benefits of AIP Juicing. Focus on ingredients rich in vitamins, minerals, and antioxidants.

Rotate Ingredients: Rotate your ingredients regularly to ensure a diverse nutrient intake and prevent the development of new sensitivities. This helps maintain a balanced and varied diet.

Include Healing Herbs: Incorporate anti-inflammatory herbs such as turmeric, ginger, and mint into your juices. These herbs not only enhance flavor but also contribute to the healing potential of AIP Juicing.

Moderate Fruit Intake: While fruits are a crucial part of AIP Juicing, be mindful of sugar content. Choose lower-sugar options and balance sweetness with vegetables to avoid excessive sugar intake.

Hydrate Well: Complement AIP Juicing with adequate water intake. Proper hydration supports overall health and assists in the detoxification process.

Mindful Portion Control: Pay attention to portion sizes. While AIP Juicing provides essential nutrients, moderation is key to prevent overconsumption of certain compounds.

Observe Reactions: Monitor your body's responses to different ingredients. If you notice any adverse reactions or sensitivities, make adjustments to your recipes accordingly.

Integrate into a Balanced Diet: AIP Juicing is most effective when integrated into a balanced and varied diet. Use it as a supplement to whole foods, ensuring you receive a comprehensive range of nutrients.

By adhering to these guidelines, you can embark on an AIP Juicing journey that aligns with autoimmune principles, fostering holistic well-being and supporting your body's unique needs. Always prioritize your individual health and listen to the signals your body provides throughout the process.

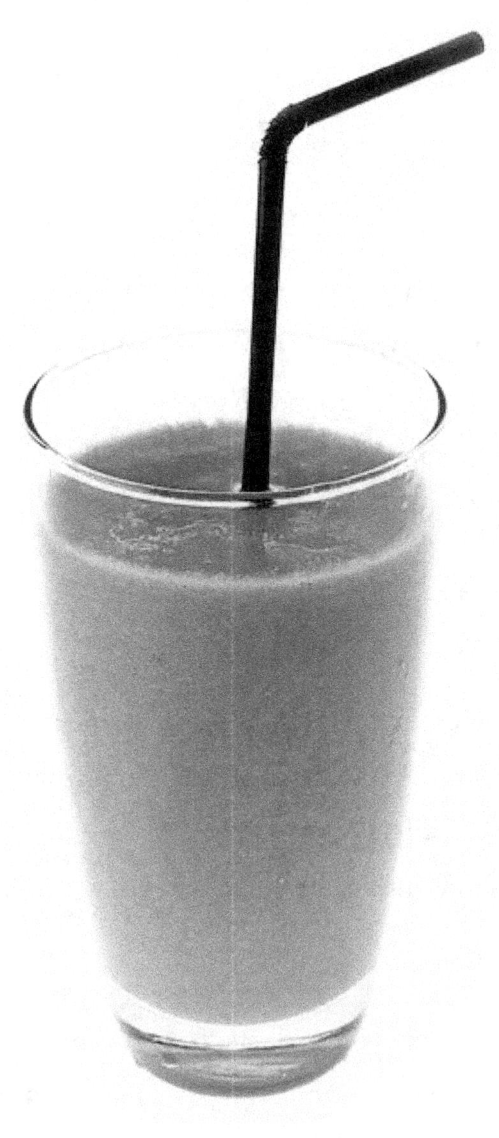

CHAPTER TWO

Autoimmune Protocol Juicing Recipes

1. Berry Citrus Blast

Ingredients:

- ➤ 1 cup mixed berries (blueberries, strawberries, raspberries)
- ➤ 1 orange, peeled and segmented
- ➤ 1/2 cucumber, peeled
- ➤ 1 tablespoon fresh mint leaves
- ➤ 1 cup coconut water

Instructions:

- ➤ Combine berries, orange segments, cucumber, mint leaves, and coconut water in a blender.
- ➤ Blend until smooth.
- ➤ Pour into a glass and garnish with a mint sprig.

Health Benefits:

- ➤ Rich in antioxidants from berries.
- ➤ Vitamin C from oranges supports immune health.
- ➤ Hydrating and refreshing.

Preparation Time: 5 minutes

2. Green Apple Ginger Zinger

Ingredients:

- ➤ 1 green apple, cored and sliced
- ➤ 1 inch fresh ginger, peeled
- ➤ 1 cup spinach leaves
- ➤ 1/2 lemon, peeled
- ➤ 1 cup filtered water

Instructions:

- ➤ Combine green apple slices, fresh ginger, spinach, lemon, and water in a blender.
- ➤ Blend until well combined.
- ➤ Strain if desired and serve over ice.

Health Benefits:

- ➤ Ginger provides anti-inflammatory properties.
- ➤ Green apple adds natural sweetness.
- ➤ Spinach offers vitamins and minerals.

Preparation Time: 7 minutes

3. Pineapple Turmeric Sunrise

Ingredients:

- ➢ 1 cup fresh pineapple chunks
- ➢ 1-inch fresh turmeric, peeled
- ➢ 1/2 cucumber, peeled
- ➢ 1 tablespoon fresh cilantro
- ➢ 1 cup coconut water

Instructions:

- ➢ Combine pineapple chunks, fresh turmeric, cucumber, cilantro, and coconut water in a blender.
- ➢ Blend until smooth.
- ➢ Pour into a glass and garnish with a pineapple slice.

Health Benefits:

- ➢ Turmeric provides anti-inflammatory benefits.
- ➢ Pineapple adds sweetness and digestive enzymes.
- ➢ Hydrating and immune-boosting.

Preparation Time: 6 minutes

4. Mango Mint Cooler

Ingredients:

> - 1 cup fresh mango chunks
> - 1/4 cup fresh mint leaves
> - 1/2 lime, peeled
> - 1 cup coconut water

Instructions:

> - Combine mango chunks, mint leaves, lime, and coconut water in a blender.
> - Blend until well combined.
> - Pour into a glass and garnish with a mint sprig.

Health Benefits:

> - Mango adds natural sweetness and vitamins.
> - Mint provides a refreshing flavor.
> - Hydrating and rich in antioxidants.

Preparation Time: 5 minutes

5. Carrot Apple Cinnamon Elixir

Ingredients:

> - 2 medium carrots, peeled and sliced

- ➢ 1 green apple, cored and sliced
- ➢ 1/2 teaspoon ground cinnamon
- ➢ 1 cup filtered water

Instructions:

- ➢ Combine carrot slices, apple slices, cinnamon, and water in a blender.
- ➢ Blend until smooth.
- ➢ Strain if desired and serve over ice.

Health Benefits:

- ➢ Carrots provide beta-carotene for eye health.
- ➢ Apple adds natural sweetness.
- ➢ Cinnamon offers a warm and aromatic touch.

Preparation Time: 8 minutes

6. Beet Berry Bliss

Ingredients:

- ➢ 1 small beet, peeled and chopped
- ➢ 1/2 cup mixed berries (strawberries, blueberries)
- ➢ 1/2 cucumber, peeled
- ➢ 1 tablespoon fresh basil leaves
- ➢ 1 cup coconut water

Instructions:

> ➤ Combine chopped beet, mixed berries, cucumber, basil, and coconut water in a blender.
> ➤ Blend until well combined.
> ➤ Pour into a glass and garnish with basil leaves.

Health Benefits:

> ➤ Beets provide antioxidants and nutrients.
> ➤ Berries contribute vitamins and minerals.
> ➤ Hydrating and nourishing.

Preparation Time: 7 minutes

7. Papaya Lime Refresher

Ingredients:

> ➤ 1 cup fresh papaya chunks
> ➤ 1/2 lime, peeled
> ➤ 1 tablespoon fresh cilantro leaves
> ➤ 1/2 cup coconut water

Instructions:

> ➤ Combine papaya chunks, lime, cilantro leaves, and coconut water in a blender.

- ➢ Blend until smooth.
- ➢ Pour into a glass and garnish with a lime wheel.

Health Benefits:

- ➢ Papaya adds natural sweetness and digestive enzymes.
- ➢ Lime provides vitamin C and a citrusy flavor.
- ➢ Hydrating and refreshing.

Preparation Time: 6 minutes

8. Blueberry Kale Kickstart

Ingredients:

- ➢ 1/2 cup blueberries
- ➢ 1 cup kale leaves, stems removed
- ➢ 1/2 cucumber, peeled
- ➢ 1/2 lemon, peeled
- ➢ 1 cup filtered water

Instructions:

- ➢ Combine blueberries, kale leaves, cucumber, lemon, and water in a blender.
- ➢ Blend until well combined.
- ➢ Strain if desired and serve over ice.

Health Benefits:

> ➢ Blueberries offer antioxidants and vitamins.
> ➢ Kale provides nutrients and a vibrant green color.
> ➢ Hydrating and nutrient-dense.

Preparation Time: 6 minutes

9. Orange Carrot Ginger Energizer

Ingredients:

> ➢ 2 medium carrots, peeled and sliced
> ➢ 1 orange, peeled and segmented
> ➢ 1 inch fresh ginger, peeled
> ➢ 1 cup filtered water

Instructions:

> ➢ Combine carrot slices, orange segments, fresh ginger, and water in a blender.
> ➢ Blend until smooth.
> ➢ Strain if desired and serve chilled.

Health Benefits:

> ➢ Carrots provide beta-carotene for skin health.
> ➢ Orange adds natural sweetness and vitamin C.

> ➢ Ginger offers anti-inflammatory properties.

Preparation Time: 7 minutes

10. Melon Mint Hydration Splash

Ingredients:

- ➢ 1 cup melon cubes (cantaloupe or honeydew)
- ➢ 1 tablespoon fresh mint leaves
- ➢ 1/2 lime, peeled
- ➢ 1/2 cup coconut water

Instructions:

- ➢ Combine melon cubes, mint leaves, lime, and coconut water in a blender.
- ➢ Blend until well combined.
- ➢ Pour into a glass and garnish with a mint sprig.

Health Benefits:

- ➢ Melon provides hydration and vitamins.
- ➢ Mint adds a refreshing flavor.
- ➢ Coconut water offers electrolytes for hydration.

Preparation Time: 5 minutes

11. Cucumber Avocado Green Goddess

Ingredients:

- 1 cucumber, peeled and sliced
- 1/2 avocado
- 1 cup spinach leaves
- 1/4 cup fresh parsley
- 1/2 lemon, peeled
- 1 cup filtered water

Instructions:

- Combine cucumber slices, avocado, spinach, parsley, lemon, and water in a blender.
- Blend until smooth.
- Pour into a glass and garnish with a cucumber slice.

Health Benefits:

- Cucumber and avocado provide hydration.
- Spinach offers vitamins and minerals.
- Parsley adds a fresh burst of flavor.

Preparation Time: 6 minutes

12. Tomato Basil Bliss

Ingredients:

- ➢ 2 cups cherry tomatoes
- ➢ 1/4 cup fresh basil leaves
- ➢ 1/2 cucumber, peeled
- ➢ 1/2 lime, peeled
- ➢ 1 cup filtered water

Instructions:

- ➢ Combine cherry tomatoes, basil leaves, cucumber, lime, and water in a blender.
- ➢ Blend until well combined.
- ➢ Pour into a glass and garnish with basil leaves.

Health Benefits:

- ➢ Tomatoes provide antioxidants.
- ➢ Basil adds anti-inflammatory properties.
- ➢ Hydrating and rich in flavor.

Preparation Time: 5 minutes

13. Sweet Potato Coconut Elixir

Ingredients:

- ➢ 1 small sweet potato, cooked and mashed
- ➢ 1/2 cup coconut milk
- ➢ 1/4 teaspoon ground cinnamon
- ➢ 1/4 teaspoon ground ginger
- ➢ 1/2 cup filtered water

Instructions:

- ➢ Combine mashed sweet potato, coconut milk, cinnamon, ginger, and water in a blender.
- ➢ Blend until smooth.
- ➢ Pour into a glass and sprinkle a dash of cinnamon on top.

Health Benefits:

- ➢ Sweet potato provides vitamins and fiber.
- ➢ Coconut milk offers healthy fats.
- ➢ Cinnamon and ginger add warmth and flavor.

Preparation Time: 8 minutes

14. Broccoli Lemon Zest Delight

Ingredients:

- ➢ 1 cup steamed broccoli florets
- ➢ 1/2 lemon, peeled
- ➢ 1/2 cucumber, peeled
- ➢ 1 cup spinach leaves
- ➢ 1 cup filtered water

Instructions:

- ➢ Combine steamed broccoli, lemon, cucumber, spinach, and water in a blender.
- ➢ Blend until well combined.
- ➢ Pour into a glass and garnish with a lemon twist.

Health Benefits:

- ➢ Broccoli provides vitamins and antioxidants.
- ➢ Lemon adds a citrusy zing.
- ➢ Hydrating and nutrient-dense.

Preparation Time: 7 minutes

15. Butternut Squash Sage Elixir

Ingredients:

- 1/2 cup roasted butternut squash, cooled
- 1 tablespoon fresh sage leaves
- 1/4 teaspoon ground nutmeg
- 1/2 cup coconut water

Instructions:

- Combine roasted butternut squash, sage leaves, nutmeg, and coconut water in a blender.
- Blend until smooth.
- Pour into a glass and garnish with a sage leaf.

Health Benefits:

- Butternut squash offers vitamins and fiber.
- Sage adds a savory and aromatic touch.
- Nutmeg provides a warm and comforting flavor.

Preparation Time: 6 minutes

16. Asparagus Cilantro Citrus Blend

Ingredients:

- 1 cup steamed asparagus

- ➢ 1/4 cup fresh cilantro leaves
- ➢ 1/2 orange, peeled and segmented
- ➢ 1/2 lime, peeled
- ➢ 1 cup filtered water

Instructions:

- ➢ Combine steamed asparagus, cilantro, orange segments, lime, and water in a blender.
- ➢ Blend until well combined.
- ➢ Pour into a glass and garnish with a cilantro sprig.

Health Benefits:

- ➢ Asparagus provides vitamins and folate.
- ➢ Cilantro adds a burst of freshness.
- ➢ Orange and lime contribute vitamin C.

Preparation Time: 7 minutes

17. Spinach Pineapple Mint Fusion

Ingredients:

- ➢ 1 cup spinach leaves
- ➢ 1 cup fresh pineapple chunks
- ➢ 1 tablespoon fresh mint leaves
- ➢ 1/2 cucumber, peeled

➢ 1/2 cup coconut water

Instructions:

➢ Combine spinach, pineapple chunks, mint leaves, cucumber, and coconut water in a blender.
➢ Blend until smooth.
➢ Pour into a glass and garnish with a mint sprig.

Health Benefits:

➢ Spinach offers vitamins and minerals.
➢ Pineapple adds natural sweetness and digestive enzymes.
➢ Mint provides a refreshing flavor.

Preparation Time: 6 minutes

18. Cauliflower Rosemary Elixir

Ingredients:

➢ 1 cup steamed cauliflower florets
➢ 1 tablespoon fresh rosemary leaves
➢ 1/2 lemon, peeled
➢ 1/2 cup coconut water

Instructions:

> ➤ Combine steamed cauliflower, rosemary, lemon, and coconut water in a blender.
> ➤ Blend until smooth.
> ➤ Pour into a glass and garnish with a rosemary sprig.

Health Benefits:

> ➤ Cauliflower provides vitamins and fiber.
> ➤ Rosemary adds a savory and aromatic touch.
> ➤ Lemon contributes a citrusy flavor.

Preparation Time: 6 minutes

19. Zucchini Basil Green Refresher

Ingredients:

> ➤ 1/2 zucchini, sliced
> ➤ 1/4 cup fresh basil leaves
> ➤ 1/2 cucumber, peeled
> ➤ 1/2 lime, peeled
> ➤ 1 cup filtered water

Instructions:

- Combine zucchini slices, basil leaves, cucumber, lime, and water in a blender.
- Blend until well combined.
- Pour into a glass and garnish with a basil leaf.

Health Benefits:

- Zucchini provides hydration and vitamins.
- Basil adds a fresh burst of flavor.
- Lime offers a citrusy zing.

Preparation Time: 5 minutes

20. Bell Pepper Carrot Turmeric Elixir

Ingredients:

- 1/2 red bell pepper, sliced
- 2 medium carrots, peeled and sliced
- 1 inch fresh turmeric, peeled
- 1/2 cup coconut water

Instructions:

- Combine red bell pepper, carrots, fresh turmeric, and coconut water in a blender.

- ➢ Blend until smooth.
- ➢ Pour into a glass and garnish with a bell pepper slice.

Health Benefits:

- ➢ Bell pepper provides antioxidants and vitamins.
- ➢ Carrots offer beta-carotene for skin health.
- ➢ Turmeric contributes anti-inflammatory benefits.

Preparation Time: 7 minutes

21. Turmeric Cauliflower Delight

Ingredients:

- ➢ 1 cup steamed cauliflower florets
- ➢ 1 inch fresh turmeric, peeled
- ➢ 1/2 lemon, peeled
- ➢ 1/2 cucumber, peeled
- ➢ 1 cup filtered water

Instructions:

- ➢ Combine steamed cauliflower, fresh turmeric, lemon, cucumber, and water in a blender.
- ➢ Blend until smooth.
- ➢ Pour into a glass and garnish with a lemon twist.

Health Benefits:

> ➤ Cauliflower provides vitamins and fiber.
> ➤ Turmeric offers anti-inflammatory benefits.
> ➤ Hydrating and nutrient-dense.

Preparation Time: 6 minutes

22. Spinach Avocado Green Elixir

Ingredients:

> ➤ 1 cup spinach leaves
> ➤ 1/2 avocado
> ➤ 1/4 cup fresh cilantro leaves
> ➤ 1/2 lime, peeled
> ➤ 1 cup coconut water

Instructions:

> ➤ Combine spinach leaves, avocado, cilantro, lime, and coconut water in a blender.
> ➤ Blend until smooth.
> ➤ Pour into a glass and garnish with a lime wheel.

Health Benefits:

> ➤ Spinach provides vitamins and minerals.

- ➤ Avocado adds healthy fats.
- ➤ Cilantro contributes a burst of freshness.

Preparation Time: 5 minutes

23. Carrot Ginger Butternut Soup

Ingredients:

- ➤ 2 medium carrots, peeled and sliced
- ➤ 1 inch fresh ginger, peeled
- ➤ 1/2 cup roasted butternut squash, cooled
- ➤ 1/2 cup coconut milk
- ➤ 1 cup filtered water

Instructions:

- ➤ Combine sliced carrots, fresh ginger, roasted butternut squash, coconut milk, and water in a blender.
- ➤ Blend until smooth.
- ➤ Pour into a bowl and warm gently if desired.

Health Benefits:

- ➤ Carrots provide beta-carotene for skin health.
- ➤ Ginger offers anti-inflammatory properties.
- ➤ Butternut squash adds vitamins and fiber.

Preparation Time: 8 minutes

24. Zucchini Broccoli Basil Elixir

Ingredients:

- 1/2 zucchini, sliced
- 1 cup steamed broccoli florets
- 1/4 cup fresh basil leaves
- 1/2 lemon, peeled
- 1 cup filtered water

Instructions:

- Combine zucchini slices, steamed broccoli, basil leaves, lemon, and water in a blender.
- Blend until well combined.
- Pour into a glass and garnish with a basil leaf.

Health Benefits:

- Zucchini provides hydration and vitamins.
- Broccoli offers antioxidants and vitamins.
- Basil adds a fresh burst of flavor.

Preparation Time: 7 minutes

25. Tomato Bell Pepper Herb Elixir

Ingredients:

- 2 cups cherry tomatoes
- 1/2 red bell pepper, sliced
- 1/4 cup fresh oregano leaves
- 1 cup filtered water

Instructions:

- Combine cherry tomatoes, red bell pepper slices, oregano leaves, and water in a blender.
- Blend until well combined.
- Pour into a glass and garnish with a sprig of oregano.

Health Benefits:

- Tomatoes provide antioxidants.
- Bell pepper offers vitamins and antioxidants.
- Oregano adds a savory and aromatic touch.

Preparation Time: 6 minutes

26. Cabbage Carrot Apple Fusion

Ingredients:

- 1 cup shredded cabbage

- ➢ 2 medium carrots, peeled and sliced
- ➢ 1 green apple, cored and sliced
- ➢ 1/2 lime, peeled
- ➢ 1 cup filtered water

Instructions:

- ➢ Combine shredded cabbage, sliced carrots, green apple slices, lime, and water in a blender.
- ➢ Blend until well combined.
- ➢ Pour into a glass and garnish with a lime wheel.

Health Benefits:

- ➢ Cabbage provides vitamins and fiber.
- ➢ Carrots offer beta-carotene for eye health.
- ➢ Apple adds natural sweetness.

Preparation Time: 7 minutes

27. Beet Berry Basil Elixir

Ingredients:

- ➢ 1 small beet, peeled and chopped
- ➢ 1/2 cup mixed berries (blueberries, strawberries)
- ➢ 1/4 cup fresh basil leaves
- ➢ 1 cup coconut water

Instructions:

> ➤ Combine chopped beet, mixed berries, basil leaves, and coconut water in a blender.
> ➤ Blend until well combined.
> ➤ Pour into a glass and garnish with a basil sprig.

Health Benefits:

> ➤ Beets provide antioxidants and nutrients.
> ➤ Berries contribute vitamins and minerals.
> ➤ Basil adds a fresh burst of flavor.

Preparation Time: 6 minutes

28. Spinach Cucumber Mint Cooler

Ingredients:

> ➤ 1 cup spinach leaves
> ➤ 1/2 cucumber, peeled
> ➤ 1 tablespoon fresh mint leaves
> ➤ 1/2 lime, peeled
> ➤ 1 cup coconut water

Instructions:

> ➤ Combine spinach leaves, cucumber, mint leaves, lime, and coconut water in a blender.
> ➤ Blend until smooth.
> ➤ Pour into a glass and garnish with a cucumber slice.

Health Benefits:

> ➤ Spinach offers vitamins and minerals.
> ➤ Cucumber provides hydration.
> ➤ Mint adds a refreshing flavor.

Preparation Time: 5 minutes

29. Bell Pepper Carrot Ginger Elixir

Ingredients:

> ➤ 1/2 red bell pepper, sliced
> ➤ 2 medium carrots, peeled and sliced
> ➤ 1-inch fresh ginger, peeled
> ➤ 1/2 cup coconut water

Instructions:

> ➤ Combine red bell pepper slices, sliced carrots, fresh ginger, and coconut water in a blender.

> Blend until smooth.

> Pour into a glass and garnish with a bell pepper slice.

Health Benefits:

> Bell pepper provides antioxidants and vitamins.

> Carrots offer beta-carotene for skin health.

> Ginger contributes anti-inflammatory benefits.

Preparation Time: 7 minutes

30. Broccoli Kale Lemon Zest Elixir

Ingredients:

> 1 cup steamed broccoli florets

> 1 cup kale leaves, stems removed

> 1/2 lemon, peeled

> 1/2 cucumber, peeled

> 1 cup filtered water

Instructions:

> Combine steamed broccoli, kale leaves, lemon, cucumber, and water in a blender.

> Blend until well combined.

> Pour into a glass and garnish with a lemon twist.

Health Benefits:

- ➢ Broccoli provides vitamins and antioxidants.
- ➢ Kale offers nutrients and a vibrant green color.
- ➢ Lemon adds a citrusy zing.

Preparation Time: 8 minutes

31. Berry Coconut Chia Pudding

Ingredients

- ➢ 1/2 cup mixed berries (blueberries, raspberries)
- ➢ 1 cup coconut milk
- ➢ 2 tablespoons chia seeds
- ➢ 1/2 teaspoon vanilla extract (optional)

Instructions:

- ➢ Blend mixed berries and coconut milk in a blender until smooth.
- ➢ In a bowl, mix the blended mixture with chia seeds and let it sit in the refrigerator for at least 4 hours or overnight.
- ➢ Stir well before serving. Optionally, add vanilla extract for flavor.

Health Benefits:

- ➤ Berries provide antioxidants.
- ➤ Coconut milk offers healthy fats.
- ➤ Chia seeds add fiber and omega-3 fatty acids.

Preparation Time: 5 minutes + chilling time

32. Cucumber Guacamole Cups

Ingredients:

- ➤ 1 cucumber, sliced into rounds
- ➤ 1 avocado, mashed
- ➤ 1 tablespoon fresh cilantro, chopped
- ➤ 1/2 lime, juiced
- ➤ Salt and pepper to taste

Instructions:

- ➤ In a bowl, mix mashed avocado with chopped cilantro, lime juice, salt, and pepper.
- ➤ Spoon the guacamole onto cucumber rounds.
- ➤ Garnish with additional cilantro if desired.

Health Benefits:

- ➤ Cucumber provides hydration.

- ➤ Avocado adds healthy fats.

- ➤ Cilantro offers a burst of freshness.

Preparation Time: 10 minutes

33. Sweet Potato Kale Chips

Ingredients:

- ➤ 1 small sweet potato, thinly sliced

- ➤ 1 cup kale leaves, torn into pieces

- ➤ 1 tablespoon olive oil

- ➤ Sea salt to taste

Instructions:

- ➤ Preheat oven to 350°F (175°C).

- ➤ Toss sweet potato slices and kale pieces with olive oil.

- ➤ Spread them on a baking sheet, sprinkle with sea salt, and bake for 15-20 minutes until crisp.

Health Benefits:

- ➤ Sweet potato provides vitamins and fiber.

- ➤ Kale offers nutrients and a crunchy texture.

- ➤ Olive oil adds healthy fats.

Preparation Time: 20 minutes

34. Apple Cinnamon Collagen Bites

Ingredients:

- ➤ 1 green apple, cored and sliced
- ➤ 1 tablespoon collagen powder
- ➤ 1/2 teaspoon ground cinnamon
- ➤ 1 tablespoon almond butter

Instructions:

- ➤ Blend apple slices, collagen powder, ground cinnamon, and almond butter in a food processor.
- ➤ Roll the mixture into bite-sized balls.
- ➤ Refrigerate for at least 30 minutes before serving.

Health Benefits:

- ➤ Apple provides natural sweetness and fiber.
- ➤ Collagen supports joint and skin health.
- ➤ Cinnamon adds a warm and aromatic flavor.

Preparation Time: 15 minutes + chilling time

35. Beet Hummus with Veggie Sticks

Ingredients:

- 1 small beet, boiled and peeled
- 1 can (15 oz) chickpeas, drained and rinsed
- 1/4 cup tahini
- 1/4 cup lemon juice
- 2 cloves garlic, minced
- Assorted vegetable sticks for dipping (carrots, cucumber, bell peppers)

Instructions:

- Blend boiled beet, chickpeas, tahini, lemon juice, and minced garlic in a food processor until smooth.
- Serve the beet hummus with assorted vegetable sticks.

Health Benefits:

- Beets provide antioxidants and nutrients.
- Chickpeas offer protein and fiber.
- Vegetables add vitamins and crunch.

Preparation Time: 15 minutes

36. Turmeric Almond Energy Bites

Ingredients:

- ➢ 1 cup almonds
- ➢ 1/4 cup shredded coconut
- ➢ 1 tablespoon honey
- ➢ 1 teaspoon ground turmeric
- ➢ Pinch of sea salt

Instructions:

- ➢ Blend almonds, shredded coconut, honey, ground turmeric, and sea salt in a food processor until a dough-like consistency is achieved.
- ➢ Roll the mixture into small energy bites.
- ➢ Refrigerate for at least 30 minutes before serving.

Health Benefits:

- ➢ Almonds provide protein and healthy fats.
- ➢ Turmeric offers anti-inflammatory benefits.
- ➢ Honey adds natural sweetness.

Preparation Time: 10 minutes + chilling time

37. Avocado Basil Zoodles

Ingredients:

- ➢ 1 zucchini, spiralized into noodles (zoodles)
- ➢ 1/2 avocado, mashed
- ➢ 1 tablespoon fresh basil, chopped
- ➢ 1/2 lemon, juiced
- ➢ Salt and pepper to taste

Instructions:

- ➢ In a bowl, mix zucchini noodles with mashed avocado, chopped basil, lemon juice, salt, and pepper.
- ➢ Toss until well combined and serve immediately.

Health Benefits:

- ➢ Zucchini provides a low-carb alternative.
- ➢ Avocado adds healthy fats.
- ➢ Basil offers a fresh and herby flavor.

Preparation Time: 8 minutes

8. Pineapple Mint Popsicles

Ingredients:

- ➢ 1 cup fresh pineapple chunks
- ➢ 1 tablespoon fresh mint leaves
- ➢ 1/2 cup coconut water

Instructions:

- ➢ Blend pineapple chunks, mint leaves, and coconut water in a blender until smooth.
- ➢ Pour the mixture into popsicle molds and freeze for at least 4 hours.

Health Benefits:

- ➢ Pineapple provides natural sweetness and vitamins.
- ➢ Mint adds a refreshing flavor.
- ➢ Coconut water offers electrolytes for hydration.

Preparation Time: 5 minutes + freezing time

9. Cabbage Wrap with Turkey and Avocado

Ingredients:

- ➢ Cabbage leaves (as wraps)
- ➢ Sliced turkey breast

- ➤ 1/2 avocado, sliced
- ➤ Fresh cilantro for garnish

Instructions:

- ➤ Steam or blanch cabbage leaves until they are pliable.
- ➤ Fill each cabbage leaf with sliced turkey and avocado.
- ➤ Garnish with fresh cilantro and secure with toothpicks.

Health Benefits:

- ➤ Cabbage provides a low-calorie wrap.
- ➤ Turkey offers lean protein.
- ➤ Avocado adds healthy fats.

Preparation Time: 15 minutes

10. Mango Tango Salsa with Jicama

Ingredients:

- ➤ 1 ripe mango, diced
- ➤ 1/2 red onion, finely chopped
- ➤ 1 jalapeño, seeded and minced
- ➤ Juice of 1 lime

> Jicama sticks for dipping

Instructions:

> In a bowl, combine diced mango, chopped red onion, minced jalapeño, and lime juice.
> Mix well and serve with jicama sticks for dipping.

Health Benefits:

> Mango provides natural sweetness and vitamins.
> Red onion adds flavor and antioxidants.
> Jicama offers a crunchy and low-calorie dipper.

Preparation Time: 10 minutes

CONCLUSION

Embracing an Autoimmune Protocol (AIP) Juicing lifestyle is not merely a dietary choice; it is a holistic commitment to nurturing your body, mind, and overall well-being.

This cookbook serves as a gateway to a journey of healing and empowerment, where vibrant health becomes an attainable reality. Through these carefully crafted recipes, we've strived to marry the principles of the AIP with the delightful experience of juicing, ensuring that flavor and nutrition coalesce seamlessly.

Each sip becomes a celebration of nourishment, offering a symphony of ingredients designed to support your immune system, reduce inflammation, and enhance your overall vitality. Beyond the tantalizing flavors and refreshing sips, this cookbook is a guide to understanding and embracing the healing power of nutrient-dense ingredients.

It underscores the significance of mindful choices in managing autoimmune conditions, fostering a deeper connection with the body's innate ability to rejuvenate. As you embark on this culinary adventure, remember that the journey to optimal health is unique for each individual.